Baking Soda Beauty & Health

74 Recipes

By: Samantha Miller

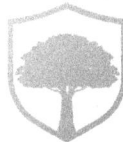

CLADD
PUBLISHING

Cladd Publishing Inc.
USA

This publication is designed to provide accurate information regarding the
subject matter covered. It is sold with the understanding that neither the
author nor the publisher is providing medical, legal or other professional
advice or services. Always seek advice from a competent professional
before using any of the information in this book. The author and the
publisher specifically disclaim any liability that is incurred from the use or
application of the contents of this book.

Baking Soda Beauty and Health: 74 Recipes
ISBN 978-1-946881-42-7 (e-book)
ISBN 978-1-946881-41-0 (paperback)

Contents

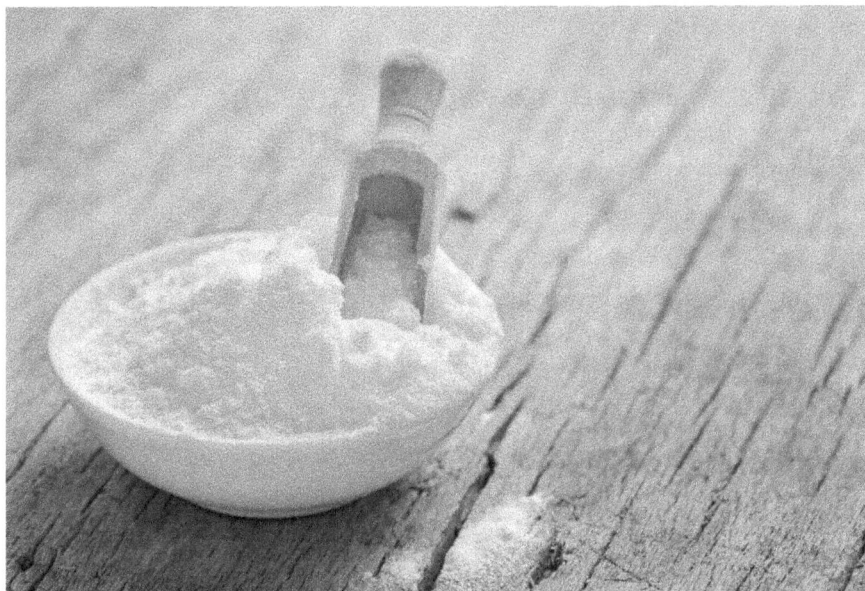

The Magic of Baking Soda

Baking Soda, also known as Sodium Bicarbonate, is a natural occurring mineral. It is absolutely one of the safest, and most versatile substances in the world.

Baking Soda in Ancient Times

The use of sodium bicarbonate, extends thousands of years into Ancient Egypt; where it was a staple in everyday life. They used it to form paint for their hieroglyphics, to clean teeth, as a powerful cleaning agent, to treat all types of wounds, and to dry out bodies for the mummification process.

ANTACID:
Baking soda has antacid properties and is beneficial to relieve acid indigestion, severe acidity and heartburn.

METABOLIC ACIDOSIS:
Beneficial in minimizing risk of metabolic acidosis in various health disorders such as diabetes, cardiovascular disorders etc. It can also provide relief of renal tubular acidosis.

DRUG POISONING:
Helps reduce poisoning caused by methyl alcohol, salicylates etc.

ANTI-ITCH:
Contains anti-itch and antipruritic properties, which help in treating various skin conditions.

IMPROVES SPORTS PERFORMANCE:
Baking soda can be beneficial in improving performance during prolonged exercise.

PLAQUE REMOVAL:

Baking soda is very effective in removing plaque from the teeth.

HYPERKALEMIA:

Hyperkalemia is ailment caused by high levels of potassium in the blood. Baking soda is effective at reducing extreme levels of potassium in the body.

KIDNEY STONES:

Baking soda helps decrease stone formation.

BLADDER INFECTIONS:

Baking soda may also help in reducing risk of bladder infections. It also eases the pain of current infections.

FEET CARE:

Baking soda inhibit yeast, fungal and bacterial growth on the feet.

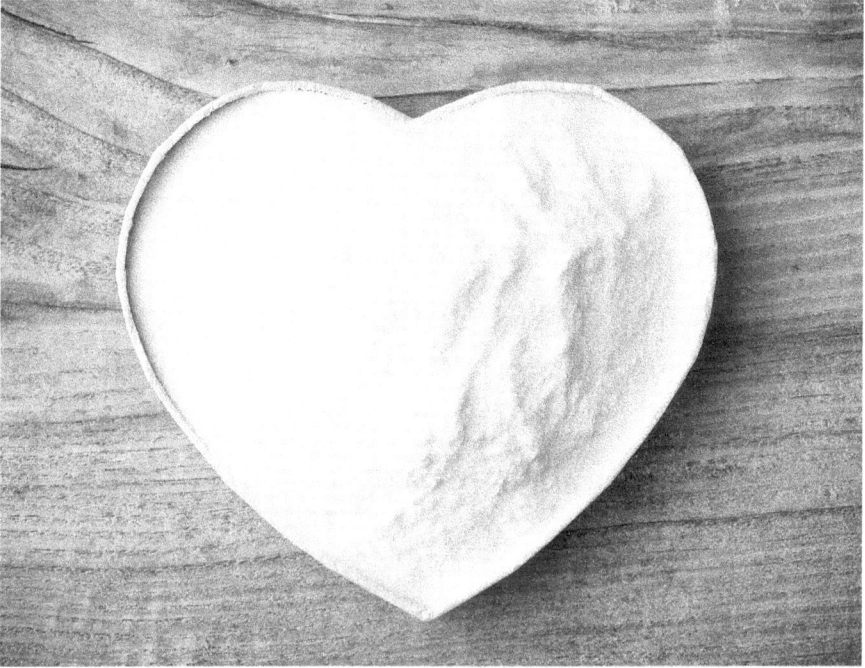

Baking Soda for Health

Your body loves sodium bicarbonate. Bicarbonate ions occur naturally in our bloodstream to aid in maintaining our acid/alkaline balance. It transports carbon dioxide from our tissues, to the lungs to be expelled.

Sodium bicarbonate is also found in our saliva as an acid reducer. The medicinal benefits go beyond comprehension; as renowned cancer and disease experts are now showing the lifesaving benefits of baking soda.

AILMENTS ITS KNOWN TO TREAT:

> ➤ Baking Soda causes food to "rise"
> ➤ Anti-fungal
> ➤ It is a natural, potent and non-toxic medicine
> ➤ High quality therapeutic agent
> ➤ Body and skin cleanser and care
> ➤ Increases your body's natural pH (alkalinity) levels
> ➤ Amazing home and vehicle cleaning solution
> ➤ Deodorizer
> ➤ And many more

Alkalinity (pH) Of the Body

If you believe your body's acidity is high, here is a quick and easy home remedy to use.

SIGNS OF HIGH BODY ACIDITY (LOW PH):

- ➤ Mucus buildup
- ➤ Joint pain
- ➤ Cold hands or feet
- ➤ Reduced sex drive
- ➤ Chemical sensitivity
- ➤ Heartburn
- ➤ Metallic taste in the mouth
- ➤ Muscular pain

Alkaline (pH) Booster

This remedy will help to balance pH levels in the body. It will also help with stomach acid and reduce acidosis.

Ingredients:

- ⅓ Teaspoons of baking soda
- 2 tablespoons of fresh lemon juice or apple cider vinegar

How To:
- Mix everything together.
- The mixture will fizz.
- Wait until the fizzing stops and add 8 ounces of water.
- Drink the mixture fast.

Alkaline Water Enhancer

Drink Alkaline water all day long and feel alive.

How To:
- Add ½ a teaspoon of baking soda to a gallon of purified water.
- Shake well.
- Enjoy at your own leisure.

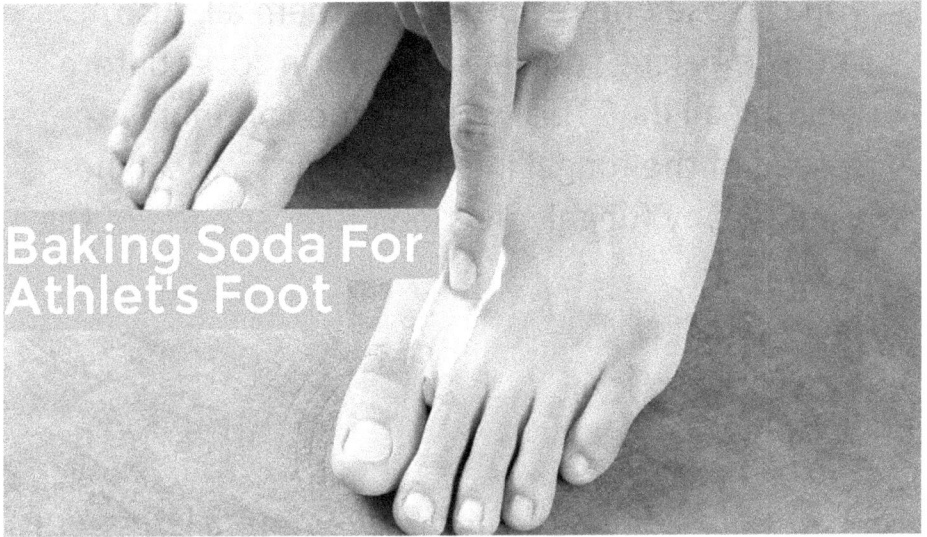

Baking Soda For Athlet's Foot

Athletes Foot – Fungal Cures

You can use one recipe, or use them all. Also, sprinkle baking soda in shoes, or in socks before wearing all day. This will stop the continuing spread of the fungal infection. This soak can be used on any fungal infection on most parts of the body.

Foot Soak

How To:

- Pour 2 liters of warm water into a large bowel or foot spa.
- Add 3 tablespoons of baking soda.
- Mix well until dissolved.
- Soak your feet for 20 minutes.
- Use a soft bristle brush on your feet and toes.
- Pat your feet dry with a clean towel.
- Moisturize with pure coconut oil.
- Use daily as needed.

Fungal Rub

How To:

- Clean your feet and pat dry.
- Mix 3 parts baking soda with 1 part water.

- Create a thick paste.
- Apply the paste on your feet and between toes.
- Let it dry.
- Wash your feet with cold water and pat dry with a towel.
- Moisturize with pure coconut oil.
- Apply 1x daily for up to 1 week.

Fungal Cream

How To:
- Pour 1 cup of vinegar and 2 cups of water into a bowl.
- Add generous amount of baking soda to form a paste.
- Mix very well.
- Apply application to both feet and between toes.
- Let it dry.
- Wash with cool water and pat dry with a towel.
- Moisturize with pure coconut oil.
- Repeat the application 2x per day for up to 2 Days.

Extreme Fungal Infection

How To:

- Combine 1 cup of pure apple cider vinegar with 1 cup of water.
- Add 2 tablespoons of baking soda.
- Mix well.
- Apply all over the feet and between toes.
- Let sit for 30 minutes.
- Wash off with cool water.
- Dry your feet with a clean towel.
- Moisturize with pure coconut oil.
- Continue 1-2x daily for 2 weeks.

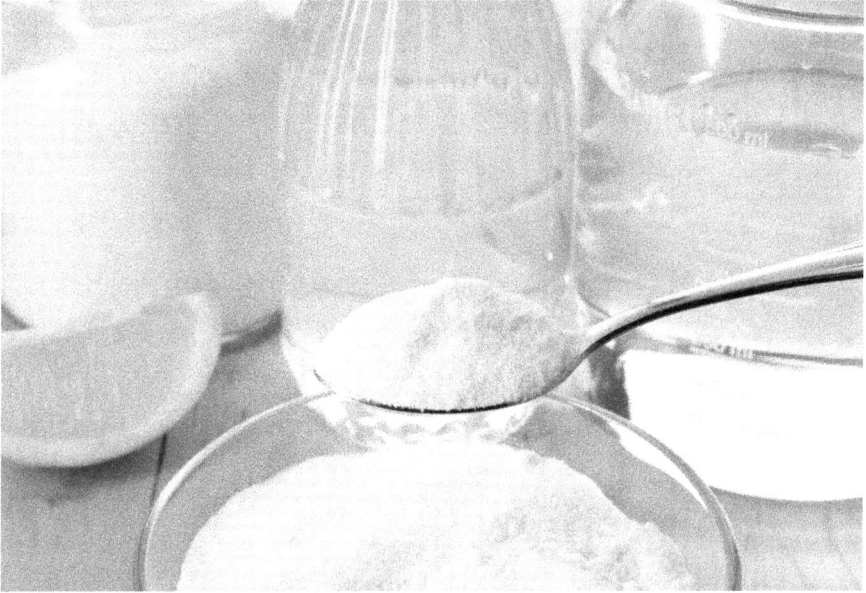

Cooking

Fluffy Morning Omelette

Make a fluffier omelet with this easy secret.

HOW TO:
- Add ½ teaspoon baking soda for every three eggs.
- Cook them as you normally would.

Tea Perfection

HOW TO:
- Use a pinch in a gallon of freshly-brewed iced tea, to take out the bitterness and prevent cloudiness.

Produce Wash

Most of our fresh produce is sprayed with some sort of chemical cocktail. It is very important to your health that you wash your fruits and vegies before consuming them.

HOW TO:
- Add 2 tablespoons of baking soda in a bowl of cool water.

- Soak them for five minutes.
- Use a wash cloth to scrub root vegetables.
- Rinse in cool water and pat dry.

Neutralize Gassy Beans

Beans can give us painful and embarrassing gas. If you are cooking them from scratch, this baking soda method will improve digestion.

HOW TO:
- Sprinkle a teaspoon of baking soda in the water when you soak beans.
- Rinse well.
- Cook as usual.

Baking Powder Substitute

Use baking soda as a substitute for baking powder by mixing with it with cream of tartar.

HOW TO:
- Mix 2 parts cream of tartar with 1-part baking soda.
- Example: mix 2 tsp cream of tartar with 1 tsp baking soda.

Fish Smell Remover

If you can't stand the way fish smells, then give it a baking soda bath to remove the odor.

HOW TO:
- Place cold water in a bowel with ½ teaspoon of backing soda.
- Soak the raw fish in the baking soda solution for an hour inside the fridge.
- Take out, give it a rinse under cool water, and pat dry.
- Cook as usual.

Tomato Sauce Acid Neutralizer

Reduce the acid content of your tomato-based recipes.

HOW TO:
- Sprinkling with a pinch of baking soda.
- Cook as usual.

Meat Tenderizer

Here is a trick for tenderizing meat that will create mouth water meat every time. It's a much healthier option than using the store-bought version.

How To:

- Rub the any kind of meat with baking soda.
- Let it rest in the refrigerator for 3 to 5 hours.
- Rinse the meat thoroughly to remove all the baking soda.
- Cook as desired.
- You can also let your meats soak in a baking soda water bath for the same amount of time.
- For smaller or thinner cut meats, soak 15 minutes to 1 hour instead.

Kick Sweet Cravings Instantly

If you're trying to avoid eating sweets, but are faced with a strong craving, then you will love this trick.

HOW TO:

- Rinse your mouth out with 1 tsp of baking soda in 4 oz of warm water.
- Gargle.
- Spit it out.
- Sugar cravings gone!

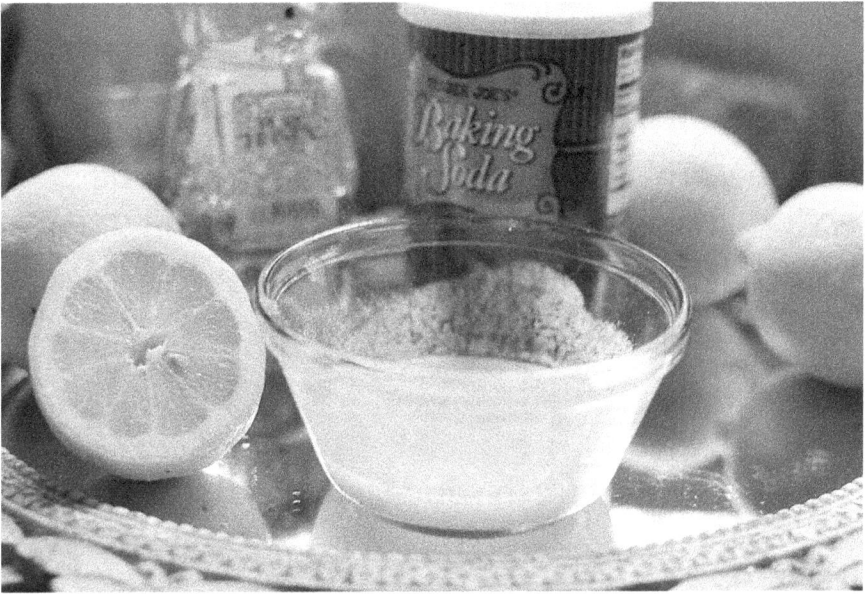

Skin & Haircare

Brightening Facemask

Having a quality facemask to rescue your skin is essential. This Lemon, Honey and Baking Soda mask will brighten your overall complexion, fade dark spots, gently exfoliates, softens skin, and is a natural antibacterial agent.

Ingredients:
- 1/2 Lemon fresh squeezed lemons (or 1 teaspoon of lemon juice from a bottle)
- 1 or 2 tablespoons of Baking Soda
- 1 teaspoon of honey

HOW TO:
- Mix lemon juice, baking soda, and honey together in a small dish.
- You should end up with a paste-like consistency. Add more baking soda to thicken.
- Wash off all makeup, dirt, and debris with your regular face wash.
- Pat skin dry.
- Apply the mask to your face and neck using circular motions.

- Leave on your skin for 5-15 minutes.
- You should feel some tingling and tightening of the mask. If your skin starts to burn, remove the mask immediately.
- Remove the mask with a lukewarm washcloth.
- Close your pores! Use the coldest water you can handle, and pat it across your face.
- Moisturize.
- Apply SPF (optional)
- Use 1x per week or less.

Damage Repair

This is an effective way to treat damaged skin. The use of the vitamin E oil penetrates deep down, while the baking soda moves oxygen through the lower layers of the skin.

How To:
- Wash the affected areas with warm water and a natural mild soap.
- Pat the skin dry.

- Combine 1 tablespoon of baking soda, 1-2 drops of water, and the content of 1 vitamin E oil capsule.
- Mix well until you get a creamy paste.
- Apply this paste on the affected areas.
- Exfoliate gently in small circular motions for 1-3 minutes.
- Wash with warm water.
- Pat the skin dry with a clean towel and apply toner and moisturizer.
- Repeat regularly.

Clear and Tighten

The antioxidants in oat flour stop the damage caused by acne and the sun. It helps the skin to retain the elasticity and firmness.

HOW TO:
- Combine 1 teaspoon of baking soda, 2 teaspoons of oat flour and 1 teaspoon of water.
- Mix to make a creamy paste.
- Apply this paste on the acne affected areas.

- Gently scrub in a circular motion for 1-2 minutes.
- Leave on for 10 minutes.
- Rinse off well with warm water.
- Repeat regularly.

Artificial tan remover

When you have experienced a self-tanning mishap, or you are just tired of waiting for the remainder to fade away, use this body exfoliator formula

HOW TO:
- One-part water to three parts baking soda.
- Gently scrub and rinse.

Razor burn soother

A razor burned bikini line can look and feel terrible. Use this hack to sooth your sensitive skin fast.

HOW TO:
- Add 1 cup of water.
- With 1 tablespoon of baking soda to form a paste.

- Allow the solution to dry on your skin (it will take about 5 minutes)
- Rinse with cool water.

FYI: Men can also use this formula for a soothing after-shave.

If it burns, stings or itches

For instant relief from bug bites, sunburn and poison ivy, this is your magic elixir.

HOW TO:
- Mix baking soda with a little water and apply it directly to the sore.
- Wash off with a warm towel after 1-3 hours.
- Reapply if you need.

Relieve Diaper Rash

This is an excellent way to relieve your baby's diaper rash naturally.

HOW TO:
- Run a warm bath.
- Add 2 tablespoons of baking soda.

- Allow your baby to soak in the tub for 10-20 minutes.

Nail scrub

It is very common to get a mild infection after pushing back, and snipping off your extra cuticles. Instead try this fabulous way to remove unwanted cuticles gently.

HOW TO:
- Create a smooth paste of: three parts baking soda to one-part water.
- Dip a nail brush into the paste.
- Rub in a circular motion over your hands and fingers.
- Rinse clean with warm water.
- Then apply nail polish as usual.

Chicken Pox – Hives – Measles

If you are suffering from chicken pox, hives, or measles then try this bath soak. It will reduce the severe itchiness and stimulates healing.

HOW TO:

- Run a warm bath.
- Put in ½ cup of baking soda.
- Soak in the tub until water cools.
- Towel off when done.

Nail Whitening

Completely mistake proof and super easy,

HOW TO:

- Pour 1/2 cup of hot water into a glass bowl.
- Add 1 tsp of peroxide.
- Add 1 tbsp. of baking soda.
- Dip your nails in and wait 1-10 minutes.
- Wash your hands and moisturize.

Sooth Sunburns

The alkaline property of baking soda soothes the skin, cools it down, relieves itching, and inflammation.

HOW TO:

- Use cool water to gently clean the affected area.
- Mix 2 tablespoons of baking soda with a little water to make a smooth paste.
- Use a cotton ball to apply the paste to the sunburn.
- Leave on for 10 minutes.
- Wash your skin with cool water and pat dry.
- Apply this type of paste regularly.

Splinter Remover

If you have a splinter that is too deep to be removed easily, this solution will force it out of your skin.

HOW TO:

- Add a tablespoon of baking soda to a small glass of water.
- Soak the affected area 2x per day.
- The splinter will be forced out within a few days.

Hand Cleanser

This natural hand cleanser will scrub away dirt and neutralize odors.

HOW TO:
- Mix three parts baking soda with one part of water to make a paste.
- Scrub hands together until clean.
- Rinse.

Chlorine Damaged Hair

After you have finished swimming, this baking soda spray will neutralize the damaging effects of the chlorine.

HOW TO:
- Add 1 tbsp. of baking soda to a small spray bottle and fill it with water.
- Spritz on wet hair.
- Shampoo and condition as usual.

Remove Dandruff

HOW TO:

- Stop dandruff by massaging your wet scalp with a handful of baking soda before shampooing.

Stop Split Ends

This will keep your hair healthy and resistant to split ends.

HOW TO:

- Mix a little baking soda with your conditioner.
- Leave in for up to 5 minutes.
- Rinse well.

Dry shampoo alternative

Use this dry shampoo alternative for crazy morning, greasy gym aftermath, and for hot summer days.

HOW TO:

- Sprinkle a few pinches of baking soda onto your roots.
- Tousle your hair.
- Then brush it to perfection.

Sprayed by A Skunk

If you or your pet has been sprayed by a skunk jump in this bath.

HOW TO:

- Add ½ -1 cup of baking soda to a hot bath.
- Soak until water becomes cool.
- Rinse off.
- Take them once per day until the skunk odor disappears.

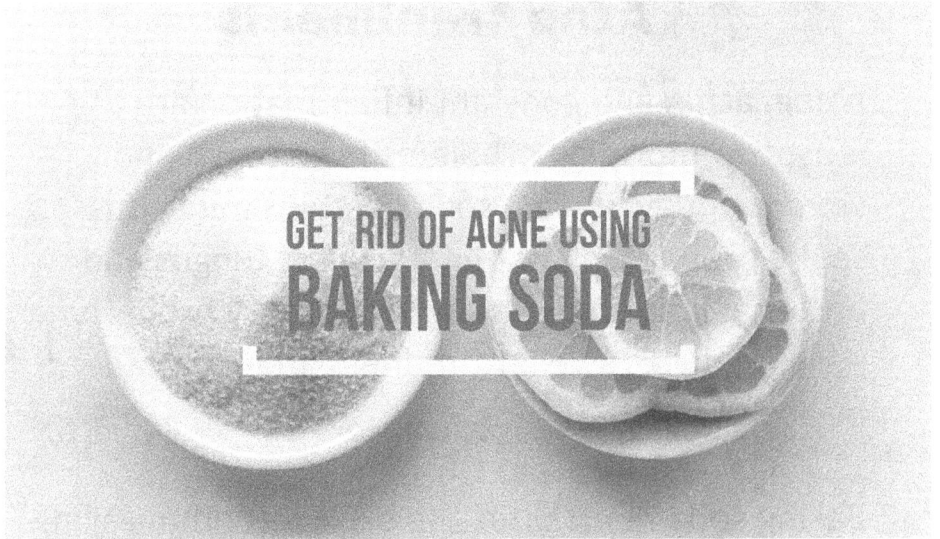
GET RID OF ACNE USING
BAKING SODA

Acne Relief

Acne Treatments

Aging, acne, and constant inflammation are the most common skin problems facing man and women today. Baking soda contains mild anti-septic properties, that fight against fungus and bacteria. It also has anti-inflammatory property which reduces swelling, redness and pain caused by acne.

Baking soda neutralizes the pH levels on the skin, discouraging the growth of bacteria. It absorbs excess oil in the skin, which leads to blackheads and breakouts. Due to its gritty nature, it contains magical exfoliating properties that effectively removes oil, dirt, dust, dead skin and so much more.

Baking soda penetrates deep into the skin, encouraging the sodium transportation into all skin cells to slow down the metabolism. By bringing more oxygen to the skin cells, your face will look and feel years younger.

Facial Acne Relief

HOW TO:

- Combine enough baking soda and water to make a creamy paste.
- Apply the paste on the acne affected areas.
- Gently massage in circular motion for 1-2 minutes.
- Let paste sit on your face for 15-20 minutes.
- Rinse paste off thoroughly with warm water.
- Repeat the process 1x per week.

FYI: Baking soda may dry out the skin. Use a good moisturizer to keep skin hydrated.

Body Acne Treatment

This process treats acne and scars on back, buttocks, chest and arms.

HOW TO:

- Add 1/2 cups of baking soda to your bath.
- Soak for 20 minutes.
- Get out and pat dry – do not rinse.
- Repeat the process regularly.

- You can also use this as a wonderful sponge bath.

Scalp Acne

This treats scalp acne and acne near the hair line. It also repairs damaged hair caused by styling gels and volumizers.

How To:
- Add 1 teaspoon of baking soda into the shampoo bottle.
- Shake the bottle well.
- Wash your hair thoroughly with this solution to treat scalp acne.
- Repeat the process regularly.

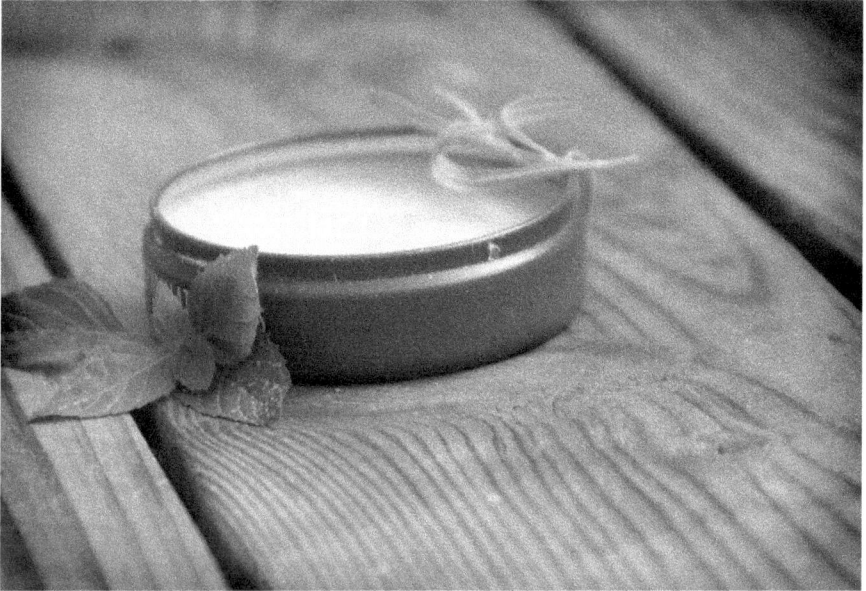

Deodorant

Most ingredients used in store-bought deodorants are toxic.

Toxic Ingredients in Store-Bought Deodorant:

- **Aluminum** –This is a metal which has been linked to breast cancer in women, and an increased risk of Alzheimer's.
- **Parabens** –Paraben exposure has also been linked to birth defects and organ toxicity.
- **Propylene glycol** – This is a petroleum based material and damages the central nervous system, liver, and heart.
- **Phthalates** – Phthalates have been linked to a variety of health issues including birth defects.
- **Triclosan** – This chemical is disturbingly classified as a pesticide by the FDA.

For All Skin Types – Even Sensitive

Making your own deodorant is not only simple, but also safe for the entire family.

Ingredients:

- 1/3 cup coconut oil.
- 2 Tbsp. of baking soda (you reduce slightly for really sensitive skin).
- 1/3 cup arrow root powder.
- 10 – 15 essential oils (You can make a plain batch, then add oils based on individual preferences).
- Small flat mason jars.

HOW TO:

- Mix the coconut oil, baking soda, and arrow root powder together in a bowl.
- Cream together the ingredients until it is similar to deodorant.
- Mix in essential oils.
- Put mixture into a small flat glass jar.
- To use simply swipe two fingers gently into the mixture and rub on your underarms.
- Wait two minutes before dressing to avoid any smearing on your clothes.

FYI: Patchouli, Sandalwood, Oakmoss, Bay, Cypress, Ginger, Black Pepper, Vanilla, Vetiver, and the citrus oils are strongly favored by men. Popular feminine essential oils are Rose, Jasmine, Geranium, Clary Sage, Sweet Orange, Lemon or Grapefruit. However, you can add any oil or combination that makes you feel happy.

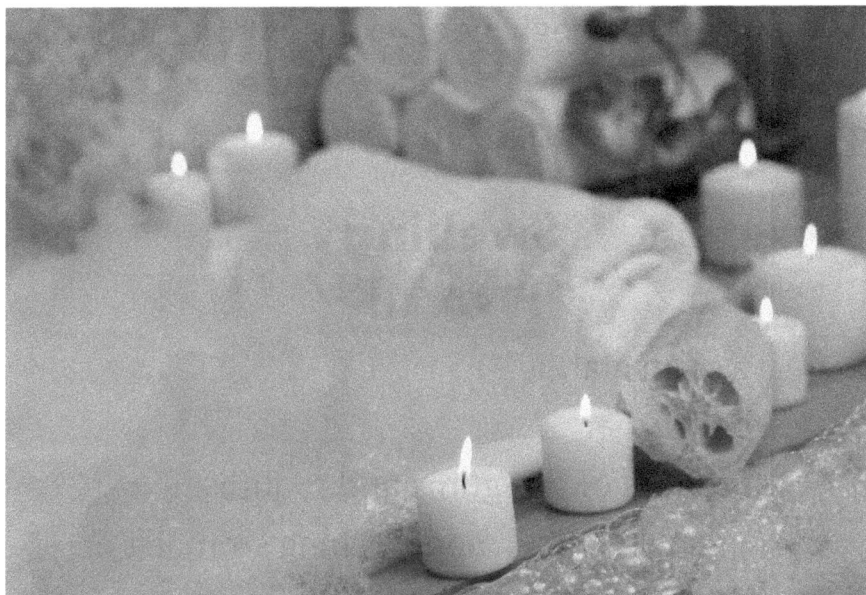

Detoxifying Baths

If you have knowingly been exposed to radiation, toxic chemicals or feel the need to detox, then try one of these great detoxifying baths.

Soreness & Swelling

Symptoms:
- swollen glands
- sore throat
- soreness of the gums and mouth
- digestive impairment (aching stomach or nausea)

HOW TO:
- Dissolve 4 cups of baking soda in a regular size tub of water hot water.
- Use more as needed if your tub is oversized.
- Get in.
- Stay in the bath until the water has cooled (approximately 45 minutes).
- Do not rinse after the bath.
- Pat with dry towel.

Radiation Exposure

Symptoms:

- exposure to environmental radiation
- x-rays
- plane flights
- or airport screenings

How To:

- Dissolve one pound of sea salt or rock salt into bath.
- Dissolve one pound of baking soda into same bath.
- Get in.
- Stay in the bath until the water has cooled (approximately 45 minutes).
- Don't add more hot water after entering the bath.
- Do not rinse or shower.
- Pat with a dry towel.
- This bath will likely make you tired.

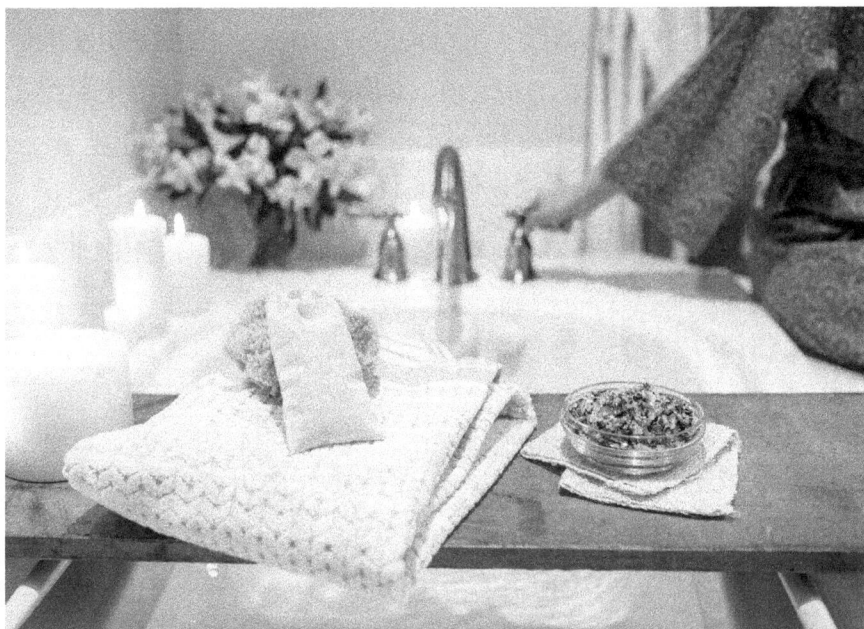

Sore Muscles & Inflammatory Bath Soaks

These bath soaks are the best remedy for reducing entire body inflammation, relieve aches and pains, muscle cramps, muscle relaxer, remove toxins, a natural emollient for your skin, and reduces lactic acid build-up. Feel the magic of body and mind!

Eucalyptus Soak

Soak in this Eucalyptus bath for purifying, oxygenating, energizing and detoxifying effects. Works wonders for general sore muscles, feet, upper and lower back pain.

Ingredients:
- 1 Cup Epsom Salts
- 1/4 Cup Sea Salts
- 1/4 Cup Baking Soda
- 3 drops each of eucalyptus essential oil and rosemary essential oil

How To:
- Mix all ingredients together in a small bowl.
- Begin filling bathtub with hot water.
- Place the mixture under the faucet as it is filling.
- Soak for at least 20 minutes.

- Do a quick rinse.
- Pat dry with a towel.
- Go bed immediately as you may become very drowsy.

Sport Soak

Refreshing salt soak for sore muscles caused by a heavy workout.

Ingredients:
- 1 1/2 cups Epsom salt
- 1/2 cup coarse sea salt or Pink Himalayan salt
- 1/2 cup baking soda
- 6-8 drops of essential oils (optional)

HOW TO:
- Mix all ingredients together in a bowl.
- Fill your bathtub water.
- Place the mixture under the faucet as its filling.
- Soak for at least 20 minutes.
- Do a quick rinse.
- Pat dry with a towel.

- Go bed immediately as you may become very drowsy.

Soothing Foot Bath

This is an excellent way to relax sore feet and reduce swelling.

HOW TO:
- Dissolve 3 tablespoons of baking soda in a tub of warm water and soak feet.
- Gently scrub.
- Soak until water begins cooling.
- Pat dry with a towel.
- Moisturize.

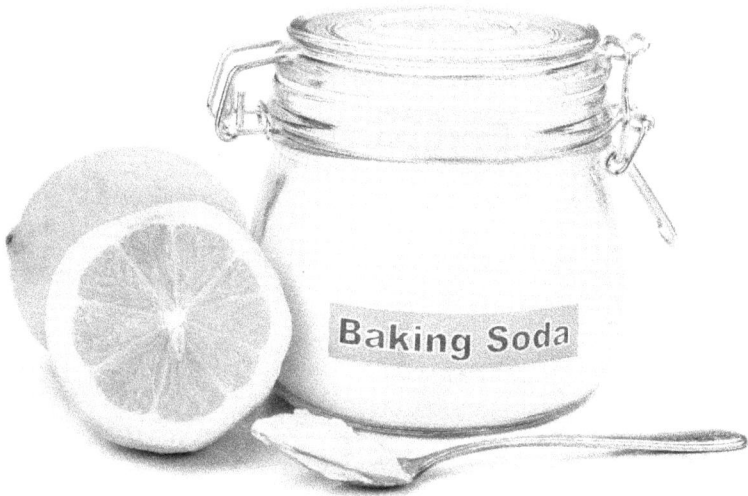

Ailments

Nasal Flush

Ingredients

- 1/2cup sea salt (real salt)
- 1/2cup baking soda
- Nasal Irrigation Bottle or Kit
- filtered water

HOW TO:

- Mix sea salt & baking soda together and store in a jar.
- Use 1/2 a teaspoon per sinus rinse.

Parasite Flush

Baking soda is effective in removing parasitic worms infesting your digestive tract.

HOW TO:

- Take this solution before bed, without food or drinks other than water.
- Dissolve a quarter teaspoon of soda in warm water and drink quickly.
- Repeat every night for three days.

Colds – Flu – Influenza

DOSAGES BASED ON AN ADULT 18+:

- **Day 1**: Take five doses of ½ teaspoon of baking soda in a glass of cool water, at two hour intervals.
- **Day 2:** Take three doses of ½ teaspoon of baking soda in a glass of cool water, at the same intervals.
- **Day 3:** Take one dose of ½ teaspoon of baking soda in a glass of cool water morning and evening.
- **Thereafter:** Take ½ teaspoon in a glass of cool water each morning until cold symptoms are gone.

Ease Urinary Pain

HOW TO:

- Mix 1 tbsp. in 32 ounces of water.
- Drink the mixture to reduce the pain of a urinary tract infection.

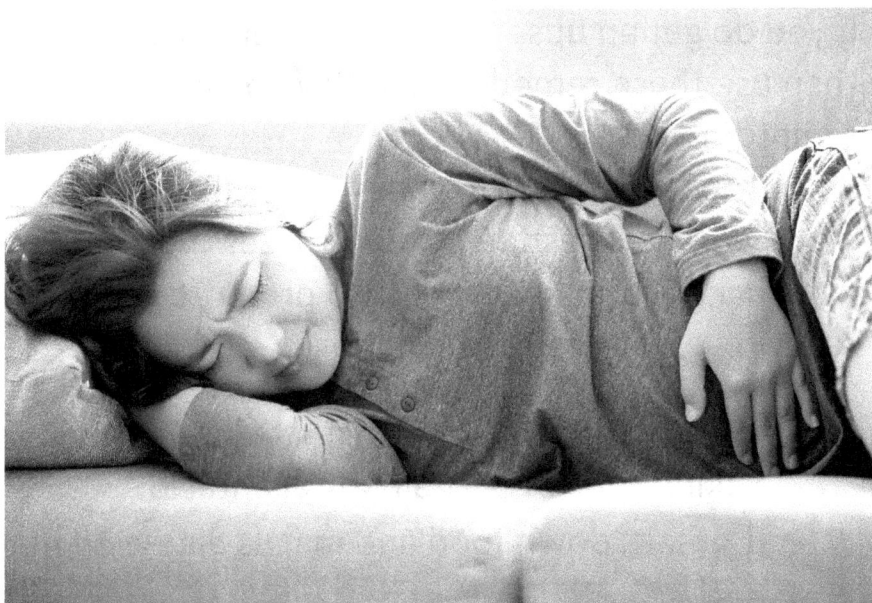

Upset Stomach

If you do get an upset stomach for any reason, then use these remedies to relieve painful symptoms.

Baking soda dissolves in water and is absorbed quickly in the intestines. It neutralizes the effects of an acidic stomach. It will also promote burping, relieving excess gas and bloating.

Baking Soda Cures an Upset Stomach:

➢ Baking soda acts as a natural antacid.
➢ It breaks down food and makes digestion easier.
➢ Baking soda restores the pH balance of the body.
➢ Baking soda relieves excess gas and bloating.

Baking Soda + Water

A simple solution prepared with water can be used; it is an easy way to cure the ailment.

Diluted Baking Soda Treats:

• Upset stomach or indigestion
• Heartburn
• Nausea
• GERD (Gastroesophageal reflux disease)

HOW TO:

- Add ½–1 teaspoon of baking soda to half a glass of water.
- Mix well to dissolve completely.
- Drink this once every 4 hours.
- This recipe is intended for adults, not children (reduce ingredients based on weight).
- Dosage should not exceed 5 teaspoons per day.

Baking Soda + Vinegar + Water

By adding the vinegar, it reduces acidity in the stomach. This is a fantastic drink that works fast.

HOW TO:

- Add 1/2 teaspoon of baking soda to small glass of water.
- Mix well.
- Now add a teaspoon of apple cider vinegar.
- The drink should begin bubbling (if it doesn't, add more baking soda and vinegar to the water).

- Let the bubbles settle down slightly before drinking.
- Drink fast.

Baking Soda + Warm + Lemon

This process helps to soothe the stomach and chest.

HOW TO:
- Add 1 teaspoon of baking soda to 1 cup of warm of water.
- Stir in a few drops of fresh squeezed lemon juice
- Mix together and drink
- Provides relief within 10–15 minutes
- Repeat every 3 hours, if upset stomach persists.

Baking Soda + Lemon + Peppermint Leaves

The peppermint leaves are uplifting and the lemon adds a touch of sunshine.

HOW TO:

- Add ½–1 teaspoon of baking soda.
- 1 teaspoon of lemon juice.
- 1-2 crushed peppermint leaves.
- ½ cup of water.
- mix it well.
- Add small ice cubes.
- Drink fast.

Foaming Water Drink

The foaming water drink is a favorite among those with a sweet tooth.

HOW TO:

- Take 2 lemons and squeeze the juice from it
- Add ½ teaspoon of baking soda and little bit of sugar or honey (to sweeten)
- Mix it well as it will foam quickly. Drink while it is foaming.

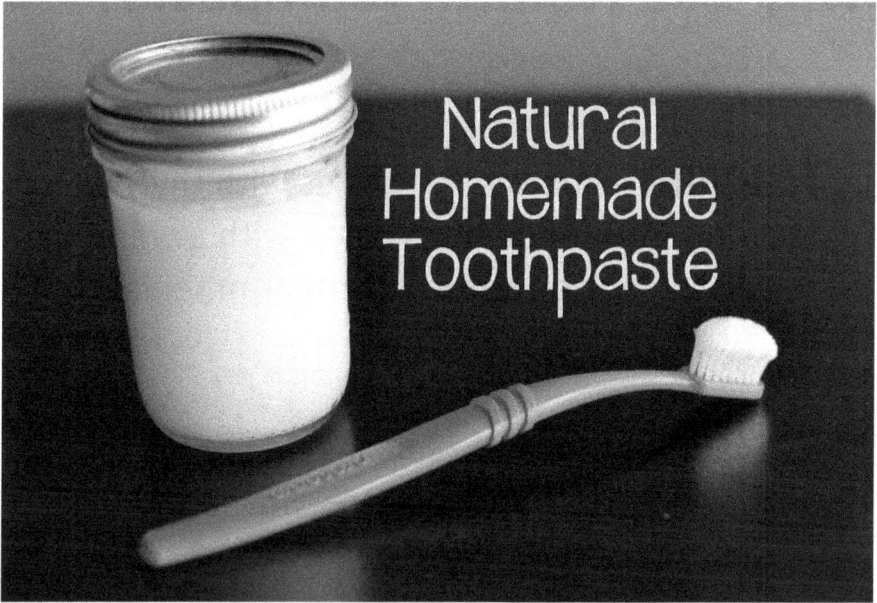
Natural Homemade Toothpaste

Toothpaste & Mouth Care

Why Use Natural Toothpaste?

Store-bought Toothpaste Ingredients:

FLUORIDE: Fluoride interferes with thyroid hormones. fluoride does come with a warning to call the poison control center immediately if ingested.

TRICLOSAN: A chemical used in antibacterial soaps and products. Triclosan was found to affect proper heart function.

GLYCERIN: Glycerin is a sweet, colorless liquid and some research says it can coat teeth and prevent them from benefitting from minerals in saliva.

SURFACTANTS: Many toothpastes contain surfactants like sodium lauryl sulfate, which gives toothpaste its foam and lather. It can cause mouth ulcers and canker sores. artificial colors/dyes or synthetic flavors.

Natural Toothpaste

Ingredients:

- 1/2 cup coconut oil
- 2-3 Tablespoons of baking soda
- 2 small packets of stevia powder
- 15 drops of peppermint or cinnamon essential oil
- 10 drops myrrh extract (optional)

HOW TO:

- Slightly soften coconut oil.
- Mix in other ingredients and stir well.
- Put mixture into small glass jars.
- Let cool completely.
- To use: dip toothbrush in and scrape small amount onto bristles.

Whitening Toothpaste

If you need to use whitening toothpaste, use this non-toxic recipe. It will whiten your teeth without experiencing the painful sensitivity that comes with store-bought tubes.

Ingredients:

- ¼ cup Calcium Carbonate Powder
- 3 Tablespoons Xylitol powder
- ¼ cup MCT oil (plus more for thinning if needed)
- Essential oils of choice (optional)

How To:

- Make sure the xylitol is finely ground and not coarse.
- Mix all ingredients by hand or with a blender until incorporated.
- Store in a glass jar and use as you would regular toothpaste.

FYI: Xylitol is naturally coarse, use the blender to make the powder fine. In case you do not know what MCT oil is, it is derived from coconut oil or palm oil. The process is unique and provides a great base for this toothpaste.

Mouthwash

This natural mouthwash kills germs, freshens breath and heals sores.

HOW TO:
- Add baking soda to a small cup of warm water
- Gargle and spit out.
- Do this 1-2 times daily.

Canker Soar Solution

This really goes to work treating painful canker sores on the lips, gums, tongue and throat.

HOW TO:
- Mix 1 tablespoon of water and 1 teaspoon of baking soda.
- Make a fine paste.
- Apply to affected areas in the mouth.
- Let sit until dry.
- Gargle with warm water until mouth is rinsed.
- It is completely safe, so do not fret if you swallowed some.
- Repeat the same process once daily.

Mouth Appliance Cleaner

Soak oral appliances, like retainers, mouthpieces and dentures, in this amazing solution.

How To:

- Dissolve 2 teaspoons of baking soda into a glass or small bowl of warm water.
- The baking soda loosens food particles and neutralizes odors to keep appliances fresh.
- You can also brush appliances clean using baking soda.

Clean Brushes & Combs

Remove oil build-up and hair product grime.

How To:

- Start by soaking brushes in 1 teaspoon of baking soda and 2 cups of warm water for 1-4 hours.
- Rinse and allow to dry.

Clean Your Toothbrush

Many people overlook the need to clean their toothbrushes. However, many disgusting things thrive on this tiny wet bristle.

How To:
- Add ¼ cup baking soda to ¼ cup water
- Let toothbrushes stand overnight.
- Rinse and use the next morning.

www.ingramcontent.com/pod-product-compliance
Lightning Source LLC
Chambersburg PA
CBHW050605280326
41933CB00011B/1993